Barefoot Strong

Unlock the Secrets to Movement Longevity

Dr Emily Splichal

DEDICATION

For those who have the courage to step out of their comfort zone and challenge the accepted.

Always push past life's challenges, fulfill your dreams and live a life full of passion.

CONTENTS

ACKNOWLEDGEMENT

I want to thank everyone who has supported and encouraged me as I pursued my dream to spread the power of barefoot training across the world. Your selfless support kept me motivated through the long flights and endless nights.

Thank you to all my Education Partners and Master Instructors from across the world who believe in my barefoot education program and the positive impact we can make as a unified profession.

Thank you to all the professionals who have attended one of my courses and have spread the power of barefoot training with your family, friends, patients and clients.   Hearing your success stories fuels my fire to continue to spread this message.

#barefootstrong

Dr Emily

1 | BAREFOOT – BEYOND RUNNING!

As a Doctor one of my favorite aspects of my job is educating and empowering patients to take their health and well-being into their own hands.

Most patient complaints could have been prevented if they had a little deeper understanding of the way in which the body moves, how forces are transferred upon foot strike and the importance of soft tissue recovery.

For the past several years *Barefoot Strong* has been a vision of mine.   I wanted a means to further spread the message of foot health, barefoot science and from the ground up programming to professionals, patients, athletes, clients and consumers across the world.

After dedicating my Master's degree towards researching the science behind barefoot training and the power of neuromuscular activation from the ground up, my approach towards Podiatry, functional movement and patient care has not been the same.

Barefoot Beyond Running

Captivated by media and the minimal footwear industry, the word 'barefoot' is often associated with running or minimal shoes.

However, when a person begins to explore and experience the power behind barefoot activation and foot to core integration, the application of 'barefoot" far exceeds that of simply running.

It is my goal to share this powerful method for restoring movement, eliminating pain patterns and giving hope to those who thought impaired movement was an acecepted part of their life.

It is time to take the word "barefoot" beyond running! Through *Barefoot Strong* it is my goal to teach the world how to become BAREFOOT STRONG!

Becoming Barefoot Strong

As I began to outline this book, I started to realized the deeper meaning behind the words BAREFOOT STRONG and what they meant to me.

I began to see that BAREFOOT STRONG means so much more than simply working out sans footwear.

To me, barefoot strong is a way of life.

It is a belief system built on the foundation of respect for the human body and the way in which it was designed to control and create the beauty of movement.

To truly become BAREFOOT STRONG, I believe that one must:

- *Accept* that the neuromuscular system is a deeply integrated network of joints, fascia, muscles and nerves which work together like a symphony providing the beauty we call human movement

- *Respect* the foot as a kinematic structure serving as the foundation to all closed chain movements

- *Appreciate* the sensitivity of the plantar proprioceptors and their role in maintaining balance, perceiving impact forces and stabilizing the lumbopelvic hip complex for human locomotion

- *Refuse* to allow the continuous damping of neuromuscular input due to footwear and unnecessary orthotics but rather welcome the proprioceptive input from the ground on which we stand.

So what does BAREFOOT STRONG mean to you?

2 | THE BARE FOOT

As the only contact point between the body and the ground, our feet play a critical role in the way in which our body controls and reacts to every upright movement.

With 26 bones, 33 joints, 19 muscles and 107 ligaments the human foot is a fascinating and complex biomechanical structure.   However the functional importance of the foot does not stop at pronation and supination.

With thousands of plantar receptors, the foot is also a proprioceptive-rich structure, containing thousands of small nerves that are sensitive to every subtle movement we make.

Our ability to walk, run or jump is all initiated through stimulation of these nerves on the bottom of the foot.

80% of our plantar proprioceptors are sensitive to vibration – Nigg et al.

I remember when I was first applying to Podiatry School and the reactions I would get from friends and family. "Feet? Why would you ever want to work with feet?"

I used to feel embarrassed to tell strangers I was dedicating my career to one of the dirtiest, and often hidden, parts of the body.

However, as I began to learn more and more about the intricate biomechanics and neuromuscular control of the foot, I found myself becoming increasingly fascinated with my profession. I began to appreciate the foot for the work of art that it is and now it is my goal to share this passion with professionals across the world.

With a passion for human movement and an internal association between movement and happiness, I began to see the foot as the gateway to our ability to experience the joy of movement.

Today, with every patient I treat it is my goal to empower them with the skills needed to maintain or restore movement at any age.

To fully tap into the skills of movement longevity there must be a deeper appreciation for the integrated function of the foot, as well as the power behind the barefoot.

The Foot, Our Foundation

Much awareness was brought to the power of the bare foot in 2009 when Chris McDougall released his New York Times Best Seller *Born to Run*. Coupled with the rise in minimal footwear such as Nike Free and Vibram FiveFingers, the barefoot running boom had coaches, runners and enthusiasts ready to learn about the importance of the plantar foot in human movement.

Considered one of the most proprioceptive rich areas of the human body, the plantar foot responds to and can actually anticipate every closed chain movement we do.

With small nerve receptors sensitive to stimuli such as texture, vibration, pressure and skin stretch, the skin on the bottom of the foot is unique when compared to skin on the top of the foot or the lower leg.

Although all skin of the human body is proprioceptive-rich, not all nerves are the same size or respond to stimuli at the same speed.

In the foot we have two sizes of nerves - *small* and *large* - with the smaller nerves being found in the bottom of the foot. Because of the smaller diameter these plantar nerves are able to send signals faster to the Central Nervous System, creating faster response times. We will explore this concept more in Chapter 5.

These smaller nerves also play an important role in quiet stance and upright stability. If you think about our daily routine of putting on socks and shoes each morning, do you ever wonder what this is doing to the input of the plantar nerves?

As soon as we put on socks, orthotics or shoes we block these highly sensitive small nerves on the bottom of the foot.

Even the most minimal "barefoot" shoe to some degree blocks these plantar receptors. So what impact does this have on our function?

Any blocking or skewing of input to the plantar nerves causes a delay in response time and creates a greater reliance on the slower, large nerves found in the ankle and lower leg.

Although this shift in proprioceptive feedback is subtle and doesn't quite result in us falling - it still has a negative impact on the way in which our foot controls and reacts to the demands of human movement. This is especially apparent as it relates to our ability to load impact forces during walking. More on this in Chapter 2.

From Mobile Adaptor to Rigid Lever

In addition to being a proprioceptive-rich structure the intricate biomechanics of foot allows us to load and unload impact forces with every step.

Often referred to as a rigid lever and mobile adaptor, the foot is not only able to adapt to uneven terrain (think hiking), but is also able to generate up to eight times our body weight in elastic forces!

The joint in the foot that unlocks this elastic power and allows functional integration between the foot and the rest of the body is known as the *subtalar joint* or STJ.

As one of the two joints in the rearfoot the STJ is formed by the talus above and the calcaneus below.

With movements including inversion and eversion, the stability of this joint dictates how we transfer forces and load potential energy between heel strike and push off.

To fully appreciate foot function and integration you want to experience the movements of the STJ.   For a video on how to move the STJ please visit www.barefootstrong.com

Experience STJ Mobility

Start by standing with your feet shoulder width apart. Roll onto the outside of your foot so that you are increasing your medial arch.   This is referred to as STJ *inversion.*

STJ inversion is associated with a rigid, stable and locked foot. This is the STJ position we want to be in when releasing energy or accelerating.

STJ inversion equals a rigid, stable and locked foot.

Now roll onto the inside of your foot so that you are flattening your arch. This is referred to as STJ *eversion*.

STJ eversion is associated with a flexible, unstable and unlocked foot. This is the STJ position in which we load energy or decelerate.

Return to the start position and now lift your heels so you are on the ball of your foot. In this position your STJ is again inverted and is locked or unloading energy. This reflects the position of our foot when pushing off or jumping. The ability to pull the STJ into inversion is critical to optimizing energy release.

Lower back down to your heels and move into a squat position. In the bottom of a squat your STJ is everted which means it is unlocked and loading energy. Although we may not see the STJ eversion in a squat, this movement of the STJ is necessary to properly load the squat and transfer energy.

STJ eversion equals a flexible, unstable and unlocked foot.

Experience Joint Coupling

As we stand up again and begin moving the foot between inversion and eversion, begin to notice the movements of your knees, hips and pelvis.

As you move the STJ do you feel how your knees and hips are rotating inward and outward?

These rotations that travel from the foot, up into the leg are referred to as *joint coupling*.

STJ eversion is coupled with internal rotation of the knee and hip and equals loading energy.

———————

STJ inversion is coupled with external rotation of the knee and hip and equals unloading energy.

———————

It is this joint coupling during foot strike that allows impact forces and potential energy to travel up the body. Although we focus on these rotations into the hip they actually continue into the trunk and thoracic spine making something as simple as walking a truly integrated movement from the foot up.

Foot Type & Function

As we move throughout our day, our foot is continuously moving between inversion and eversion.

When we are not moving, the ideal position for the STJ is in what's called *neutral*. I often refer to the STJ as a seesaw with inversion on one side, eversion on the other and neutral in the center.

It is this balanced neutral position where we want our foot to sit when relaxed. Any deviation between this centered neutral position and we get compensation patterns and compromised movement. This deviation from a neutral STJ is also where we get our different foot types.

Introduction to Foot Types

Because our baseline foot posture dictates much of our function understanding your foot type is important.

When it comes to foot types many people have heard the terms over-pronation and over-supination. Many shoes stores now offer gait assessments or foot screens to determine foot type.

Although these are good attempts at guiding the customer towards more appropriate footwear, there is still a lot of confusion and misinformation on the market.

With a heavy push towards orthotics and motion controlled shoes, the general public is led to believe that our feet by-design are weak and in need of supportive devices. Unfortunately, this could not be further from the truth!

When I teach foot types to my patients and in my courses, I rarely refer to feet as over-pronated or over-supinated. Instead I look at the individual joints, particularly the STJ, when describing foot type.

What is your Foot Type?

To determine your STJ position you will need a partner or way to take a picture of the back of the foot.

Standing with your feet shoulder width apart and heels directly behind the toes, take a picture of the back of the heels where the Achilles tendon inserts into the calcaneus.

Make sure that the picture is taken parallel to the ground and at eye level with the feet. For a video on how to properly determine foot type please visit www.barefoostrong.com

The Neutral Foot

If your Achilles insertion is straight or you do not notice any concavity on the inside or outside of the heel, then your STJ position would be considered *neutral*.

This is the ideal foot type as far as its ability to properly load and unload impact forces, as well as its ability to switch between a mobile adaptor and a rigid lever.

To maintain optimal foot function the neutral foot would want to incorporate daily foot recovery and foot strengthening exercises. More on this in Chapter 7.

The Inverted Foot

If your Achilles insertion is curved towards the inside of the foot or there is a concavity on the inside of the heel, then your STJ position would be considered *inverted.*

An inverted foot by design is functionally more rigid than the other foot types. This means that as the demand to load impact forces or the need to manipulate uneven terrain increases, the inverted foot may functionally not be able to keep up.

The result?   An increased risk of impact-related injury including stress fractures or Achilles tendonitis.

Due to the rigidity of the inverted foot, daily foot mobility is key for optimal foot function.   Again this will be reviewed in Chapter 7.

The Everted Foot.

The final foot type and STJ position is the *everted* foot. In this foot type the Achilles insertion is curved towards the outside of the foot or there is concavity on the outside of the heel.

This foot type will function almost opposite that of the inverted foot. With STJ eversion being synonymous with an unlocked foot, the everted foot generally is unstable, flexible and has a hard time becoming a rigid lever or releasing potential energy.

The ability to rapidly unlock and lock the foot is necessary for peak performance - especially in sports or movements that require rapid acceleration or change of direction.

People with an everted foot typically are at greater risk of experiencing diffuse foot pain, knee pain and low back pain. Due to this instability this foot type is probably the most common associated with custom orthotics.

Due to the instability of the everted foot, daily foot strengthening is key for optimal foot function. More on this in Chapter 7.

Foot to Core Sequencing

The final fascinating fact about of the human foot is that it is deeply integrated with the stability of our core.

In movement science there is a saying "proximal stability for distal mobility". What this means is that in order to walk, run, kick, jump etc., our core (often referred to our powerhouse) must be stable (strong) enough to transfer forces.

Despite all the research supporting the interconnection between feet and core, it was not until recently that people began to appreciate this interconnection.

There are 2 primary ways in which our feet and core are integrated:

1. Co-Activation Patterns
2. Fascial Integration

Co-Activation Patterns

Co-activation means that the firing of one muscle leads to a simultaneous firing of another muscle. This simultaneous muscle firing, also known as a co-activation, could be in a neighboring muscle or it may be in a muscle further down the chain.

From a functional perspective, co-activation firing patterns lead to faster stability allowing more efficient movements and improved performance.

One such co-activation pattern that many people are familiar with or may appreciate is one that relates to core strength.

To be strong in the core requires much more than simply having a strong six pack. Core strength is the result of all abdominal muscles working together and firing as a unit. Activation of the pelvic floor leads to a co-activation of the transverse abdominals which leads to further co-activation of the multifidi, internal obliques and so forth.

Understanding the above co-activation pattern for the core is why most people have moved away from doing simple crunches and moved towards integrating more planks, push-ups and wood chops into their core training program.

Similar to the core activation pattern above, there is a co-activation pattern between the feet and core. I refer to this co-activation pattern as the *foot to core activation cascade*.

To fully appreciate the foot to core activation cascade we must first have a deeper understanding of hip and core anatomy.

Deep Hip Stability

The reason I put so much emphasis on hip stability is because I believe the hip is the driver of all core stability during closed chain movements.

During walking, the forces generated by foot contact travel directly up the leg and into the deep hip.

Within milliseconds of foot contact our hip must prepare for the single leg stability needed during midstance. Any delay in hip stability will result in improper knee and foot alignment which presents as IT band syndrome, patellofemoral pain syndrome or ankle sprains, to name a few.

To stabilize fast enough there is another co-activation cascade that occurs in the deep hip.

Do you know which muscles start this deep hip co-activation cascade?

If you guessed the glutes you are close, but we need to go much deeper into the hip joint.

There are a group of muscles known as the *deep lateral rotators* or deep six rotators that surround the hip joint. Acting much like the rotator cuff of the shoulder, these deep muscles suction the femoral head into the hip joint providing the first layer of deep hip stability.

The deep lateral rotators provide reflexive hip stability needed for single leg stance.

If we were to continue down our co-activation cascade, these deep lateral rotators lead to co-activation of the pelvic floor which leads to co-activation of the diaphragm, psoas major and so forth until our glutes activate and we have established optimal hip and core stability.

Only once we have established the above deep hip to core stability are we prepared to transition into a single leg stance and transfer forces.

So how do we tie this back to the foot?

It is actually the foot that drives this deep hip co-activation cascade!

The foot drives the deep hip reflexive stability needed during closed chain movement.

Foot to Core Activation Cascade

Step 1. Foot Activation (Short Foot)

The foot activation exercise that research has demonstrated increases deep hip and pelvic floor activity is referred to as *short foot*.

Originally introduced by Czech Physiatrist Dr. Vladimir Janda, short foot is probably my favorite foot exercise.

This powerful foot activation exercise specifically targets one of the small muscles in the foot known as the *abductor hallucis*.

As it's name suggests the abductor hallucis abducts the hallux or big toe, keeping the great toe joint in proper alignment. In addition to it's biomechanical benefits it is also associated with neuromuscular co-activation of the deep lateral rotators and pelvic floor.

Activating Short Foot

To perform short foot exercise start by standing *barefoot* on both feet, but focus your attention on one foot at a time.

Find your foot tripod that is under your 1st metatarsal head, 5th metatarsal head and heel. Lift your toes, spread them out and place them back down onto the ground.

Notice the even body weight distribution under your foot and how it feels to be in full contact with the ground. There is an energy that comes from the floor that you can feel when you are in full contact with the ground.

I usually do not talk too much about this in my workshops but this concept is called *Earthing*. If you are curious to learn more I recommend Googling this concept for more information.

To activate short foot push the tip of your big toe down into the ground. If toes 2 – 5 also push down that is okay. As you push the big toe down into the ground you should feel the muscles of the arch engage. Begin to notice the ball of your foot lifting off of the ground and an increase in your medial arch.

Hold short foot for 10 seconds before releasing and trying it on the other foot. To see a video demonstration of how to perform short foot please visit www.barefootstrong.com

Some additional cues that can assist in engaging short foot is to imagine pushing the foot down into the ground as if you are rooting yourself. Some people find it beneficial to imagine drawing the heel towards the ball of the foot.

Still not feeling short foot? It can be more difficult for someone with flat feet or a bunion to engage short foot. Thankfully there are a few modifications to assist these individuals.

Achieving Short Foot with Flat Feet

The reason why having a flat foot makes it difficult to engage short foot as to do with the instability of this foot type. One of the jobs of short foot is to pick up the medial arch so if you have a low arch or no arch, the engagement of the abductor hallucis will be difficult.

A trick that I like to use with these individuals is to first de-rotate the lower leg before activating short foot. If you have a flat foot start by externally rotating the lower leg with will lift the heel bone into a more neutral position.

From here, lock in short foot with the big toe and heel bone. To see a video demonstration of achieving short foot in a flat foot, please visit www.barefootstrong.com

Achieving Short Foot with a Bunion

Similarly, when a person has a bunion they may find it difficult to engage short foot. In a bunion deformity the abductor hallucis has been pulled from the side of the great toe to under the foot, shifting the pull of this muscle.

A trick to increase the short foot activation with a bunion is to either use kinesiology tape or athletic tape to pull the toe into a proper position. Or you can also use a product called Bunion Bootie www.bunionbootie.com that will hold the toe neutral.

Step 2. Deep Hip Activation

After you have the hang of short foot it is now time to start integrating it with co-activation of the deep hip stabilizers and pelvic floor.

Start by standing on one foot with a slight bend in the knee. Because short foot creates a locking mechanism to the foot and leg you always want to with a slight bend in the knee. Doing short foot on a fully locked out knee will create torque to the knee joint and meniscus.

Always do short foot with a slight bend in the knee to avoid torque to the meniscus.

Make sure the foot is straight with the heel directly behind the toes. Find your foot tripod, spread the toes and start to find your short foot activation.

Hold short foot for 10 seconds and then release.

Hold short foot again for 10 seconds, but this time start to focus on the deep hip and pelvic floor. As you engage short foot you should start to feel muscles firing in the hip and core.

To increase the intensity actively engage your pelvic floor and transverse abdominals while holding short foot. In Chapter 7 we will go into additional exercises you can do before integrating short foot to get better core activation.

Step 3. Glute Engagement

Finally it's time to start integrating the glutes or more superficial muscles with this foot activation cascade.

To feel how your glute engagement dramatically increases with a strong foot to core connection we need to go back into our short foot position.

Start back in the single leg stance with the foot straight and knee slightly bent. Do not activate short foot yet, but start to move in and out of a couple single leg squats. They do not have to be deep squats but merely a slight knee flexion and extension.

Hold your next repetition on the bottom phase of the squat. It is here that you want to activate short foot. As you hold the bottom of the squat push your big toe down into the ground. You should feel that your deep hip and core lock in, establishing deep hip stability.

Keep holding short foot as you press out of the squat, engaging your core and glutes. As you repeat this exercise you should begin to notice that the degree of glute engagement is increasing.

What you are experiencing is how our mobilizers, or in this case glutes, are designed to function. Optimal strength of our glutes requires a stable foundation from which they contract against. It is the deeper stabilizers that establish this foundation.

Optimal glute function requires
deep hip stability.

This means for optimal function our deep stabilizers must fire before our mobilizers. To do so our stabilizers must anticipate our movement patterns. We will find out that this anticipation is achieved through barefoot training!

Delayed Foot to Core Sequencing

Since before we were even walking, this foot to core activation cascade was already pre-programmed in our nervous system. Unfortunately over time and with age, we begin to lose this reflexive co-activation and stabilization between the foot and core.

One of the biggest factors contributing to this delayed activation cascade is footwear! In Chapter 3 we will begin to explore the negative impact footwear has on the way in which our body responds to impact forces and transfers energy. We will learn how footwear eventually will make us all inefficient movers who are dependent on supportive devices.

Fascia & Foot Function

The final area of foot function that we will focus on in this chapter is related to fascia.

You do not need to be a Doctor or Physical Therapist to appreciate the importance of fascia in human movement.

For the average gym goer, fascia is typically associated with foam rolling or trigger point release. It is important to note that the function of fascia far exceeds that of joint mobility

This connective tissue web envelopes our muscles, tendons and bones, controlling and integrating every move we make. Whether we are turning our head or opening a door, this fascial network is playing a role in these movements.

Our fascia is organized in what are referred to as *fascial lines*. You learn more about these fascial lines by visiting www.anatomytrains.com and checking out the book Anatomy Trains by Thomas Myers.

We have a posterior fascial line that runs from the bottom of the foot, up the calves, through the hamstrings, all the way up to the top of the skull.

Similarly we also have a lateral fascial line that runs from the bottom of the foot, along the side of our lower leg, up the iliotibial band (ITB), all the way up through the skull.

These fascial lines created an integrated network through which tension is generated, stability is achieved and forces are transferred.

If we bring it back to the foot and our foundation, most of these fascial lines pass through or originate in the bottom of the foot.

There is one fascial line in particular which is specifically responsible for deep joint stability and is the foundation of foot to core sequencing. This fascial line is the *deep front line*.

Starting in the bottom of the foot, the deep fascial line runs up the lower leg, up the inner thigh and to the pelvic floor. When we engage short foot we are technically activating this deep fascia line and re-enforcing foot to core stability.

In the next chapter we are going to take a closer look at the gait cycle, how the body absorbs impact forces and the important role barefoot activation and this fascial connective tissue web has on energy transfer.

3 | UNDERSTANDING IMPACT FORCES

When we were born and first entered the proprioceptive rich environment our nervous system was developing into one that would one day be able to control upright movement.

Unique about Homo sapiens is that we are upright bipedal beings that are able to balance and manipulate terrain on two feet.

Introducing Movement Efficiency

When we begin to look at walking and human movement it is important to understand that our nervous system was designed to preserve energy and find homeostasis or balance within our body.

To preserve energy is to move *efficiently*. Movement efficiency is one of the key components to movement longevity.

Although you may not think about movement efficiency during your daily routine, your nervous system is seeking to conserve as much energy as possible.

If we take for example walking.

Walking is merely a series of falls onto a single leg stance in which foot contact is followed by a rapid peak in ground reaction forces. Because our body seeks to conserve as much energy as possible it is actually designed to use these impact forces as the potential energy to take the next step.

Impact forces provide the energy needed for human movement.

Although this is the way our body was designed to move, very few people train with this understanding. Due to medical misinformation impact forces are often associated with overuse injures such as shin splints and stress fractures.

What we will soon find out is that it is not the impact forces that are the cause of the injury; it is actually a flaw in how our body perceives and responds to these impact forces.

Our Perception of Impact Forces

I often ask my patients and professionals in my workshops how they think we perceive impact forces.

The most common answer I get is - *pressure*.

Although we associate impact and force with pressure we actually perceive impact forces as *vibrations*. The vibrations causes by ground reaction forces are set at a certain frequency that our muscles are programmed to respond to.

Impact forces are perceived as vibrations.

So how does our body perceive these vibrations?

When it comes to our perception of vibrations we must go back to the foot. As the only contact between the body and the ground it makes sense that our perception of impact forces must begin with the foot.

In Chapter 2 we discussed plantar mechanoceptors that were sensitive to stimuli - including vibrations.

What is quite interesting is that 80% of our plantar receptors are sensitive to vibration - making this the most important stimuli in which our foot uses to control movement.

Studies have shown that it is our ability to detect vibrations which allows us determine if a surface is hard, soft, slippery etc. In addition we use vibrations to maintain balance as well as use these vibrations as potential energy when we walk.

Innate Loading Response

So once we perceive these incoming vibrations, how does our body then damp or absorb the vibrations so that we do not get injured?

After being sensed by the skin on the bottom of the foot, the vibrations enter our muscles. All muscles of the body are housed in compartments or bundles surrounded by a fascial sheath.

In the foot there are nine muscle compartments and four in the lower leg- each designed to respond to these vibrations.

As the vibrations enter the muscle compartment the muscles respond by contracting isometrically. If you are not familiar with an isometric contraction, it is similar to the contraction we do in a plank or if we hold the bottom of a squat. Isometric means that force is being generated but no joints are moving.

Vibrations are damped through isometric contractions.

To further grasp this concept of isometric contractions and vibrations, I often give an analogy to a tuning fork.

When you strike a tuning fork it begins to vibrate. One of the quickest ways to stop the tuning fork from vibrating is to touch it.

The act of touching the tuning fork is analogous to the isometric contractions of our muscles.

In addition to the damping of vibrations, another important reason why our muscles contract isometrically is to protect the long bones of our feet and legs.

Isometric contractions create a splint effect, preventing the bones from vibrating or bending upon impact. If the muscles do not contract isometrically and the bones begin to vibrate, stress fractures can occur.

When I treat a patient with stress fractures or shin splints I know immediately that their foot muscles were not contracting fast enough to adequately splint their bones. This can be from a variety of reasons but having weak muscles in the feet is the most common cause.

Weak foot muscles can lead to increased risk of stress fractures.

Delayed Damping

So if weak muscles of the feet and lower leg are associated with a delayed damping response and increased risk of impact injuries - what causes this foot weakness in the first place?

Two of the biggest contributors I see for delaying the loading response are *shoes* & *fatigue*.

As soon as we put on our shoes we block the thousands of small receptors on the bottom of the foot.

Any barrier between the plantar foot and the ground, including socks, will cause a delay in the loading response.

Although this delay is small it doesn't mean it is insignificant. Remember that when we walk impact forces peak within less than 50 milliseconds. So even a small millisecond delay overtime will have a negative effect.

Negative Impact of Shoes

In addition to delaying the loading response, Nigg et al. has shown that cushioning and extra support in shoes has been actually decreases the strength of our feet. This gradual increase in foot laziness puts us at high risk for impact related injures.

Imagine being in thick supportive shoes for over 30 years and how deconditioned the foot must become?

As a society we have become dependent on shoes and orthotics to do all the work versus tapping into our natural neuromuscular response system.

In Chapter 4 we will further explore how footwear has negatively impacted our movement patterns as well as our ability to transfer impact forces efficiently – thus interfering with our movement longevity.

Negative Impact of Fatigue

The second way in which our loading response can be delayed is due to fatigue. Fatigue is one of the biggest contributors to injury, and not just impact injuries. An increased incidence of ACL tears and low back pain or disc herniation has been associated with increased fatigue.

We have all at one time experienced the fatigue in which I am referencing. You are at the end of a ski run or you are almost at the finish line of a race. Your legs are heavy and your actions are a little clumsy.

The cause of this clumsiness or slowed reaction time is - yes fatigue - but it's actually the build up of lactic acid in our muscles.

Lactic acid is the by-product of anaerobic metabolism and is often associated with muscle soreness.

Research has since disproven this theory and we now know that muscle soreness is caused by micro-tears and inflammation in our muscles secondary to overload and tissue stress.

What lactic acid is associated with is the fatigue that we were describing above. As the name suggests, lactic acid is an acid which means it changes the pH of our muscles - making the environment acidic.

Since our muscles can only contact in a specific pH range, this increase in acidity leads to impaired or delayed muscle contractions.

In Chapter 7 we will show you how warming-up barefoot and doing our *Barefoot before Shod Program* can greatly decrease your risk of injury by offsetting fatigue.

Warming up barefoot can offset muscle fatigue and decreases your risk of injury.

Impact Forces as Potential Energy

So let's say you properly damp impact forces through isometric contractions. What does your body then do with these impact forces?

After properly damping impact forces your body converts these vibrations into what's called *potential energy*.

This potential energy will later be used as *elastic energy* to drive our next step.

To further understand the concept of potential energy and human movement, we must go back to the fascia we discussed in Chapter 2.

If you remember, fascia is the connective tissue web that surrounds our muscles, tendons and bones making our body one big interconnected network.

I want you to think of the muscle compartments that are surrounded by fascia almost like the skin or sheath that surrounds sausage. As the muscle contracts isometrically, the fascial sheath is able to slide and move with the joints.

As the fascia moves with the joints it is being stretched or loaded like a rubber band or a spring. This stretch of the fascia increases its potential energy.

Similarly to the elastic energy released when we let go of a stretched rubber band, as soon we begin to lift our heel the potential energy of our fascia changes into elastic energy and our leg is recoiled forward.

With each successive step, the ability to load and unload our fascia increases until eventually our connective tissue is able to generate *twice* as much elastic energy relative to the amount of impact forces that were encountered.

This doubling of our elastic energy is referred to as the *catapult effect* and is the mechanism through which basketball players are able to jump over 3 feet high!

It is the loading of our facia and tendons which allows us to double the forces entering the body.

Deceleration through Eccentrics?

This concept of isometrics challenges how we originally thought impact forces were absorbed and energy was transferred.

Previous theories on impact forces and overuse injuries relied much more on eccentric muscle contractions and joint mobility. The research of Dr Nigg from the University of Calgary has since challenged this concept.

Nigg's *Muscle Tuning Theory* supports the anticipatory isometric contractions upon foot strike and is the current model from which overuse injuries are assessed.

In line with this theory, if impact forces are being loaded in less than 50 milliseconds, the most efficient way to prevent overuse injury is to anticipate these forces and actually begin loading the vibrations before the foot even contacts the ground.

This is ultimately the science behind barefoot training and will be the focus of Chapter 7.

Barefoot training creates anticipatory muscle contractions leading to faster loading responses.

Foot Type & Impact Injury Risk

So we understand that impact forces are a natural and beneficial part of human movement but what if you still find yourself susceptible to impact forces?

There are two main ways that you can reduce impact forces during walking:

1. Understanding your foot type
2. Changing the way you strike the ground

In Chapter 2 we discussed the different foot types.

By now you should have determined if your foot type is rigid (inverted), unstable (everted) or neutral.
If you do not remember your foot type then I recommend referencing Chapter 2 and taking the *Foot Type Test*.

Remember that an inverted foot is structurally more rigid. This means that upon foot strike it does not have the flexibility, or time, to unlock and load impact forces.

Due to it's rigidity this foot type is susceptible to impact related injuries such as Achilles tendonitis, stress fractures and plantar fasciitis.

An inverted foot is structurally more rigid making it more susceptible to impact-related injuries.

To reduce risk of impact injury, the inverted foot should focus on foot mobility (see Chapter 7) as well as try to change the way in which the foot contacts the ground in what's referred to as walking conscious.

Conversely, in an everted foot that is structured unstable, the ability to stiffen the foot upon impact is impaired. This lack of rigidity in the foot also increases the risk of impact injures but through a different mechanism.

An everted foot is unstable making it difficult to stiffen upon foot contact.

Our foot needs to be balanced between a rigid lever and a mobile adaptor. To reduce risk of impact injury, an everted foot should focus on foot strengthening especially to the small muscles of the feet (see Chapter 7).

If you are lucky enough to have a neutral foot you are still susceptible to impact injuries however this risk is more dependent on your movement patterns and not your foot type. General foot mobility and strength is recommended for this foot type.

Walking Conscious

Next to breathing, walking is the second most common subconscious movement we do daily. Just like breathing, it is these subconscious patterns that are often taken for granted.

By becoming conscious of how hard your foot strikes the ground or the degree of dorsiflexion upon heel strike, you can vastly alter the magnitude of impact forces entering the body.

When re-teaching my patients how to walk consciously, I tell them to find the rhythm in each step. Feel how the foot strikes from the outside of the heel, rolls to the center of the foot and then off of the digits.

The fluidity of this motion begins with a subtle heel strike that should mimic walking on ice or almost flatfooted. Interestingly the less dorsiflexion you have in the ankle upon heel strike, the lower the impact forces you will encounter.

Another great tip I like to give my plantar fasciitis and Achilles tendonitis patients is to dorsiflex the great toe upon heel strike. The dorsiflexion of the great toe increases the stiffness of foot, allowing better transfer of vibrations. This is one of the reasons why impact injury rate is so high in flip-flops or thongs.

If you have never had your gait assessed I recommend asking a friend or colleague to film you walking or you can even set it up yourself.

Because walking is so subconscious simply watching your gait on video brings many of the asymmetrical movement patterns to the forefront.

For videos on how to assess gait please visit www.youtube.com/ebfafitness

4 | FROM BAREFOOT TO SHOD

As we embrace this increased awareness towards the importance of feet and barefoot training we must remember that we still live in a shod society, surrounded by a concrete jungle gym.

The Rise in Overuse Injuries

Over the past several years in my office I've seen an increase in patients with impact-related injuries including stress fractures, shin splints and Achilles tendinitis.

What's surprising is that a majority of these overuse injuries are not happening in my runners and dancers -but rather in everyday people who are getting injured simply walking to work!

I think it says something about our current relationship with impact forces if patients are getting stress fractures walking 20 blocks to their office.

Why this increase in impact injuries?

What has changed in our ability to load impact forces? And what can we do to reduce our risk of overuse injuries during everyday activity?

Introducing Surface Science

All surfaces provide a certain frequency of vibrations when contacted by the foot. With the optimal frequency around 15-20 Hz our neuromuscular system is designed to create a reflexive response to this input.

It is these vibrations that provide the energy we need to take the next step and therefore our ability to match this frequency is important in the reduction of injury risk.

The science of surfaces is built around the concept of vibrations and potential energy. Whether we are considering a fitness studio floor or a gymnastics floor, the way the surface vibrates is intentional and specific for performance.

The repetitive movements of a step class or Zumba require a forgiving surface that will match the vibrations caused by thousands of foot to floor contacts in a 60-minute class.

Similarly, the high velocity tumbling pass of a gymnast requires a surface that will match impact forces exceeding 10x body weight in less than 150 milliseconds.

This relationship between the foot and ground must be mutually beneficial meaning that as impact forces are transmitted into the body they must also be transmitted *into* the surface.

Anticipation of Impact Forces

Research by Nigg et al. has shown that as we walk, by the 3rd or 4th step our nervous system has already pre-programmed a response to match the degree of impact forces being encountered.

It is as if the foot begins to anticipate and predict the degree of impact forces during activity.

This concept of anticipation is referred to *pre-activation neuromuscular responses* and is a key component to movement efficiency and ultimately movement longevity.

Now although this may seem like a big word or complex theory, in simple terms it means that after enough repetitions your body begins to create muscle memory or subconscious movement patterns in response to impact forces.

Any dancer, gymnast or even musician who has practiced a routine or song over and over again is essentially establishing pre-activation muscle patterns into their subconscious.

Eventually what happens is the muscles begin to initiate a response to movement before the joint has

moved. This anticipation contraction is in our deep stabilizers that were covered in Chapter 2.
With walking this pre-activation response is simply our foot and ankle muscles stiffening and contracting isometrically before foot strike.

Nigg's research has found that these pre-activation responses are the only way in which the foot can load impact forces fast enough – especially when they are entering the body between 50 and 150 milliseconds.

Altered Anticipation of Impact Forces

So if our nervous system is designed to anticipate impact forces, what happens if the impact forces we are anticipating doesn't match the actual degree of impact forces we encounter?

Have you ever stepped off a curb and expected the ground to be higher, only to land with a jarring impact?

This is an example of a mismatch between the body and ground, relative to anticipated impact forces.

Now imagine doing this with every step you take. The result is overuse impact-related injuries.

Another great example that further builds an appreciation for this pre-activation theory has to do with Cirque du Soleil dancers.

In Dr Nigg's latest book Biomechanics of Sports Shoes, he references a case study involving the Cirque du Soleil dancers in Los Angeles.

Due to the meticulous training of the dancers, very few injuries are reported by Cirque du Soleil. Several years ago when they got a new stage the dancers started complaining of Achilles tendonitis and plantar fasciitis (two impact-related injuries).

Dr Nigg went to the training facility in L.A. and examined the stage. Nigg noticed that there were support beams throughout the underside of the stage – beams which would alter the vibration frequency when a dancer would land in this area.

According to the pre-activation theory if the dancers' nervous system was expecting a certain degree of vibrations but they happened to land on the stage over the beam there would be a different vibration frequency and a mismatched loading response.

Nigg recommended that the beams be removed and the stage made into one consistent compliancy. This uniform surface compliancy would allow accurate anticipation of impact frequency.

What was the result?

All the dancer's injuries went away!

I now approach all my patients and athletes with this theory in mind and can start identifying the change in surfaces that are associated with their injury pattern.

A mismatch between anticipated vibration frequency and loading response leads to injury.

I encourage you to begin to look at injury patterns relative to surfaces, adaptation and anticipation of impact forces.

Unnatural Surfaces Impair Efficient Movement

Outside of sports and performance, how do the surfaces we spend a majority of our days encountering impact injury risk?

Most of the surfaces we encounter on a daily basis, including concrete, tile or marble, do not transmit vibrations well. Impact on these surfaces is still present but instead of vibrations being transmitted through the surface *and* through the body - all vibrations are transmitted proximally through the body.

This increase in forces through the body alters the vibration frequency and therefore impairs the accuracy of the anticipated loading response.

The result?

These excess vibrations are carried over from the soft tissue into our bones and tendons - presenting as stress fractures or Achilles tendonitis.

So what can we do to reduce our risk of impact injuries on these unnatural vibrations? Keep reading to find out!

Introduction to Footwear

Not only does today's society require movement on unforgiving, unnatural surfaces but it also requires us to wear shoes.

The evolution of footwear is quite fascinating, with it's origin dating back to 40000 BC. By the 12th and 13th Century footwear was seen as a status statement that was the beginning of footwear shifting away from function and towards fashion.

In the 1950's with the advance in industrial materials such as rubber and synthetic cloth, the first athletic footwear began to hit the market. Paralleled with the increased awareness towards health and fitness we began to see the first aerobics shoe by Reebok and the first running shoe by Nike.

By the 1970's Nike was at the forefront of athletic and running footwear. Just like today, in the 1970's runners were experiencing a high rate of overuse impact-related injuries. As a result of this high injury rate Nike designed what we now associate with traditional athletic shoes – extra cushion and a heel toe drop.

Initially cushion in shoes was added on the theory that the cushion would absorb some of the impact forces, taking the stress off of the tissue and decreasing the risk of injury. However, this was not the case.

Studies by Nigg et al. have shown that the presence of cushion in shoes actually *increases* impact forces.

The reason for this increase in impact forces has to do with barefoot science. As we put on shoes, socks, orthotics we begin to block the plantar

receptors, skewing our perception of how hard we are striking the ground.

Our response? Strike the ground harder.

Cushion in shoes has been associated with an increase in impact forces.

___

To further reduce a runner's injury risk a heel toe drop was introduced. With the average heel toe drop being 12 – 14mm or ½ inch, the concept behind this feature was to take tension off of the Achilles tendon.

Although a heel toe drop takes tension off of the Achilles tendon it ultimately impairs the foot's ability to load impact forces. When our foot is placed in a heel toe drop the ankle plantarflexes and the STJ inverts – making the foot more rigid.

In a neutral or inverted foot this STJ inversion locks the foot impairing its ability to evert and load impact forces. In an everted foot this heel toe drop could actually be seen as beneficial as it puts the foot in a more stable position.

This is why understanding different foot types and how each functions is important to achieving movement efficiency.

A heel toe drop can impair the foot's ability to unlock and load impact forces.

Footwear Future

With the rise in popularity in barefoot running, minimal shoes are now a billion dollar sector within the footwear industry.

Whether Nike, Vibram or New Balance is your go-to brand there a few key features to all minimal shoes.

First feature is *lack of support* or cushioning. The minimal sole creates a more flexible shoe that requires the natural strength of the foot to properly load and unload impact forces. After gradually transitioning to this footwear many people have noted improved function and decreased joint pain.

In addition, the lack of cushion allows a more accurate perception of impact forces entering the body and therefore creates more conscious movement patterns and faster loading responses.

All foot types can benefit from lack of support and cushioning, some may require a little longer transition period or extra foot strengthening to reduce the risk of injury. More on this in Chapter 7!

The second feature of minimal shoes is the *lack of a heel toe drop*. You may have heard the term "zero drop" which means that there is a 0mm drop between the toes and heel.

It's important to note that not all minimal shoes are a true zero drop, and this is okay. Transition minimal shoes have a heel toe drop of 4mm – 8mm while zero drop shoes have a heel to drop of 0mm – 3mm.

Which shoe is best for you?

When determining which minimal shoe is best for you I always recommend basing this on your foot type, injury history and workout or sport.

In a flat foot I suggest doing a more transition shoe such as the Nike Free 5.0. The slight heel toe drop keeps the STJ in a slight inversion that allows better foot stability.

Similarly in a high arched rigid foot which may have a history of Achilles tendonitis I also recommend the transition shoe. The slight heel toe drop keeps the tension off of the Achilles tendon but allows a better loading response when compared to traditional shoes.

In the neutral foot or the person with no injury history true zero drop shoes can be worn. Remember that even the most neutral foot is still susceptible to injury and therefore foot recovery and foot strengthening is important. More on this in Chapter 7!

Surviving in a Shod Society

So we know that footwear and unnatural surfaces is a part of our everyday life. What can be done to survive in today's society?

Step 1 – Keep the feet strong

Strong feet are the first line of defense against impact-related injuries. Our ability to stiffen the foot upon heel strike will ensure vibrations are controlled and do not enter into the bone.

Short foot and other barefoot exercises are the best way to keep the feet strong. Chapter 7 will introduce all the exercises needed to stay barefoot strong.

Step 2. - Keep the feet flexible

The ability to unlock the foot is a necessary step in the loading of impact forces. Foot flexibility occurs in the form of fascial tissue therefore daily massage or trigger point release to the bottom of the foot is key.

Remember that flexibility should not be confused with instability. A flat foot that is inherently unstable must still focus on foot recovery and fascial flexibility for the proper transfer of forces.

Step 3 - Foot to core integration

The faster we can stabilize the core, the more efficient we will be at transferring forces. This reflexive core stability must be achieved from the ground up.

The exercises we learned in Chapter 2 and will review in Chapter 7 are key to optimal function in an

unnatural environment. These co-activation patterns must be trained weekly to keep them active and properly stored in the subconscious.

5 | BAREFOOT BABY BOOMERS

You have probably read at least a dozen articles advocating the benefits of protecting cognitive function as we age. From exercise to crossword puzzles, there are many ways to keep your brain sharp as you age.

When it comes to nerve health, how much do you think about *peripheral* nerve health with age?

Our ability to maintain an active lifestyle and participate in the hobbies we enjoy is just as dependent on a strong and healthy peripheral nervous system as it is to cognitive function.

By having a deeper understanding of how our nervous system functions and the impact of age on neuromuscular control, we can make a few simple changes which will ensure years of efficient movement and movement longevity.

The Nervous System

Comprised of both the Central Nervous System (CNS) (brain & spinal cord) and Peripheral Nervous System (PNS) (nerves & axons), our nervous system is responsible for coordinating voluntary and involuntary actions.

Our PNS is a complex network of spinal nerves and nerve plexuses branching out from the spinal cord. Traveling distally from the spinal cord, it is the peripheral nerves that are sensitive to outside stimulation entering the body.

These peripheral nerves make up the plantar receptors of the foot that are sensitive to input signals that go back up to the CNS. The CNS processes these input signals and sends an action signal back down to the PNS resulting in controlled, precise movements.

Movement Accuracy

To improve the accuracy and efficiency of each movement, our neuromuscular system is controlled by either a feed forward or feedback system..

Feed forward responses (aka pre-activation responses) are based on previous experiences or past muscle activation patterns.

These responses are stored in an area of the brain referred to as the cerebellum – and occur before the completion of the movement.

An example of a feed forward response would be activating the ankle stabilizers before foot contact, while a form of training that falls under feed forward would be barefoot training.

Conversely, feedback responses (aka reactive responses) allow our neuromuscular system to adjust to errors, and auto-correct throughout a given movement.

An example of a feedback response would be activation of ankle stabilizers when walking on an uneven terrain and a form of training that falls under feedback would be a wobble board or Bosu.

When considering the importance of neuromuscular responses, the rate at which the information is processed translates to more precise movements and movement efficiency.

Between feed forward and feedback responses, the faster of the two is feed forward.

Age & Input Accuracy

Where the concept of neuromuscular control, movement efficiency and aging come together is through the accuracy of input signals as dictated by the peripheral nervous system.

The more accurate the information coming in, the more precise our movements will be.

If we were to imagine someone of an older age, we typically picture someone who is more frail and timid in his or her movements. We may note a delay in the correction of movement errors and often associate this delayed correction with an increased risk in falls.

With falls being one of the biggest concerns as we age, instability and decreased control can often be attributed to an aging peripheral nervous system. So is there anything that can be done to protect the nervous system as we age so that we can maintain the movement accuracy of our younger years?

Or must we succumb to the often inevitable process of an aging neuromuscular system?

The good news is there is absolutely something you can do to protect your peripheral nervous system from the aging process. It is called *neuroplasticity through barefoot science.*

These may sound like big words, so to better understand this concept let's continue exploring the peripheral nervous system - specifically as it relates to the plantar foot.

Plantar Proprioceptors

What's unique about the PNS and the foot is this is where the smallest nerve branches exist. Divided into both sensory and motor nerves, cadaver studies have shown that 3 times as many branches of the tibial nerve (foot nerve) provide sensory function versus motor function.

The peripheral nerves that have a *sensory function* in the skin are referred to as *cutaneous nerves* or in the bottom of the foot they are our *plantar cutaneous receptors* (aka plantar mechanoceptors).

These small plantar cutaneous nerves are responsible for processing information such as texture, skin stretch, vibration, deep pressure and light touch - all of the stimuli which allows us to maintain upright stance, manipulate uneven terrain and absorb impact forces.

Our ability to detect surface compliancy and impact forces is heavily dependent on vibration detection. The importance of this sensory input is demonstrated by the fact that 80% of our plantar receptors are sensitive to vibration!

80% of our plantar foot receptors are sensitive to vibration

If we go back to aging and the accuracy of input information for precise and controlled movements, the importance of vibration detection is of upmost importance.

So how does aging affect our ability to detect vibration?

Studies have shown that as we age, our ability to detect vibration input decreases. From decreased plantar receptor density to increased input threshold, by the time we are age 70 our plantar foot requires twice the stimulation to create the same response!

Despite this astounding fact very few fall reduction programs or senior fitness programs involve barefoot training or exercises to protect the peripheral nerves.

This means that we need to take it upon ourselves and do everything we can to ensure accurate vibration input is entering our plantar receptors.

Footwear & Impaired Vibration Input

One of the greatest inhibitors of vibration input are the shoes we love. Regardless of their fashion and functional benefits, footwear is not a natural feature of our nervous system or environment.

Our nervous system and the bare foot were not designed to decipher impact forces through footwear and cushion.

This concept is now readily accepted within the running and minimal footwear industries but hasn't made its way into senior health or the orthopedic shoe market.

So in addition to altering our footwear, is there anything else we can we do to offset the aging peripheral nervous system and ensure years of movement longevity?

Below are some of the best tips for maintaining a vibrant peripheral nervous system that should be integrated into everyone's barefoot strong lifestyle.

Tips for Movement Longevity

Tip #1 – Keep blood sugar under control

Although we typically associate elevated blood sugar levels with diabetes, we can all experience fluctuations in our blood sugar levels.

Elevated glucose in our blood stream is toxic to our peripheral nerves. Any excess blood sugar is quickly converted into a free radical called *advanced glycation end products* or AGEs.

These AGEs cause a demyelination of the peripheral nerves causing a disruption in signal transport.

In addition the formation of AGEs stimulates an increase in oxidative stress and an up-regulation in pro-inflammatory markers.

Or simply stated elevated blood sugar levels (even in a non-diabetic) causes aging and degeneration of peripheral nerves (with the foot nerves going first!).

Watching diet and the glycemic index in food is an important first step in the management of blood sugar levels.

In addition a vitamin I often recommend to my patients which enhances blood sugar control is *Benfotiamine*.

Benfotiamine is an active form of B1 and acts by inhibiting the deoxidation of sugar or glycation.

Tip #2 – Consider Nerve Protective Vitamins

When I was in Graduate School a big part of my focus was on vitamin supplementation and diabetic peripheral neuropathy.

Having spent so much time researching this topic I became a firm believer in the benefits of the appropriate vitamins in protecting nerve health as we age.

Everyone can benefit from nerve protective supplements – especially if we consider that elevated blood sugar levels (even in a non-diabetic) can start to damage our peripheral nerve function.

Vitamin #1 – L-Methyl Folate

Folate means folic acid – but this is not your mother's folic acid!

L-methyl folate is the activated form of folic acid that has been shown to increase nerve growth factor. When taken over a period of 6 months studies have shown an increase in epidermal nerve fiber density (or in other words more plantar cutaneous nerves.

This vitamin also goes by the FDA approved supplement Metanx.   To learn more please visit www.metanx.com

Recommended dosage: 1000 ug X 3 times day

―――――――

Vitamin #2 – Acetyl-L-Carnitine

Acetyl-L-Carnitine is another powerful nerve protective supplement.

Acetyl-L-Carnitine has been shown to decrease painful nerve symptoms, as well as increase vibratory sensation.

Remember that we maintain balance and absorb impact forces based on our ability to detect vibration so this is extremely beneficial as age!

Recommended dosage: 500mg x 2 times day

―――――――

Vitamin #3 – R-Lipoic Acid

This is probably my favorite supplement!

Touted as one of the most powerful anti-oxidants, alpha lipoic acid has been shown to improve microcirculation to peripheral nerves while decreasing oxidative stress.

A key point about alpha lipoic acid is that it must be taken in the R-lipoic acid form as the "R" form is the one that is biologically active (vs. "S" form).

Recommended dosage: 600mg x 1 time day

Tip #3 – Cardiovascular Exercise

Cardiovascular exercise has many benefits, one of which is related to peripheral circulation. The vascular system, just like the nervous system, is very intelligent meaning that if there is a loss in circulation to one area of a muscle the vascular system will create what's called *collateral circulation* (or in other words form new blood vessels).

This is why cardiovascular exercise is beneficial for those with peripheral arterial disease.

So just like the collateral circulation formed in muscles, our vascular system can create new micro-vascular pathways to our *nerves*. The more blood and oxygen to our nerves the healthier they are!

Tip #4 – Myofascial Release

When I have a patient with idiopathic nerve symptoms I often include myofascial work into their recovery program.

Our complex network of superficial and deep fascia is intertwined with just as complex of a network of arteries, veins and peripheral nerves.

As our peripheral nerves course from the spine down to the foot it is only inevitable that they may get "stuck" or "sticky" at some point.

From muscle adhesions to a loss in fascial flexibility, inflexibility can often impede nerve conduction.

Just like when you sleep on your arm and wake up with it tingling, to a smaller degree this is what's happening to our peripheral nerves when they get caught in fascial tissue.

I often recommend to my patients to release their plantar foot, up the back of the calf to the hamstrings and into the glutes and piriformis.

For those with nerve symptoms this should be done daily.

Tip # 5 – Go Barefoot!

This one pretty much goes without saying!

If our small nerves are on the bottom of the foot we want to keep them sensitive and awake through frequent barefoot stimulation.

Our nervous system is plastic – which means that it can be shaped, challenged and molded based on the stimuli it encounters.
Conversely, if you do not stimulate your peripheral nervous system and stay in thick supportive shoes everyday – slows the sensitivity of your nerves will begin to weaken, fade and atrophy.

Whether your barefoot routine includes vibration training, standing on different textures or simply walking around your home barefoot – daily barefoot stimulation is enough to keep these small nerves on point!

Want to kick it up a notch?

Workout barefoot!

6 | FASCIA & FOOT FUNCTION

Since the earliest stages of my career I had a fascination with the science of aging. Blame it on my mom for giving us kids vitamins as birthday and Christmas presents, I have many teenage memories of spending hours reading about the anti-aging benefits of different supplements.

To satisfy this continual curiosity, in 2007 I joined the American Academy of Anti-Aging Medicine (A4M) and attended some of the most cutting edge conferences on the topic of aging. From break through anti-aging cosmetics to innovative cancer therapies, the science revealed at these conferences was years ahead traditional Western medicine.

Surrounded by Plastic Surgeons and Dermatologists, most attendees didn't understand why a Podiatrist and Movement Specialist would attend these conferences. I would explain to other Doctors that just how they use anti-aging medicine to prevent collagen degradation in the face - I too use these anti-aging secrets to protect collagen degradation. In anti-aging movement instead of focusing on the collagen in the face I focus on the collagen of the fascia and myotendinous system.

Through my association with the American Academy of Anti-Aging Medicine I quickly learned that collagen, whether it is in the skin of the face or the fascia of the foot, ages through the same process. A process known as - *glycation*.

Collagen in Skin, Fascia and Tendons

Collagen, the main element found in connective tissue, provides the structural foundation to skin, fascia and tendons.

The soundness of these collagen units is determined by the stability of hydrogen bridges and covalent bonds referred to as *crosslinks*.

Crosslinks in collagen (fascia) provide strength and stability to the tissue.

Although crosslinks provide strength and stability, excessive or what are called *non-specific crosslinks* create stiffness and a lack of elastic recoil in the connective tissue. It is these non-specific crosslinks that we often call fascial adhesions.

These non-specific crosslinks are formed through a process known as *glycation*, which occurs in the presence of excessive glucose.

We described the formation of AGEs in the previous chapter. The interaction of AGEs with tissue (fascia or nerves) is called glycation.

Glycation & AGEs

So what exactly is glycation and how is it associated with elevated blood sugar?

Due to the complexity of this process we will review it again.

Elevated or excessive sugar found in the blood stream spontaneously reacts with proteins forming a free radical known as *advanced glycation end products* or AGEs.

These AGEs are responsible for forming non-specific crosslinks in collagen resulting in stiffer, non-elastic tendons and fascia.

The stiffer the connective tissue (collagen) the increased risk of micro tearing during dynamic movement.

Although micro tearing is beneficial to building muscle mass and strength, micro-tears in our connective tissue is not so advantageous.

Studies have shown that micro-tears in connective tissue are repaired with Collagen Type III vs. the normal Collagen Type I.

Collagen Type III is characterized as less elastic and stiffer when compared to Collagen Type I. This creates a repetitive micro-trauma cycle and eventual tissue degradation we know as tendonosis.

Since fascial tissue is the foundation to efficient movement, ensuring this connective tissue stays flexible and elastic is a key component to movement longevity.

So what can we do to prevent the formation of AGEs and non-specific crosslinks in our collagen?

Preventing Collagen Aging

Tip #1 Tight glycemic control

This probably goes without saying. If elevated blood sugar levels set off the chemical reaction called glycation then avoiding blood sugar spikes is obviously important.

If you have trouble controlling your blood sugar levels through diet and exercise consider the use of supplements such as Benfotiamine. This was mentioned in the previous chapter however we will go into a little bit more detail.

A 2005 study demonstrated decreased formation of AGEs in diabetic patients with a daily dose of 300mg Benfotiamine.

As an active form a Vitamin B1, Benfotiamine acts by inhibiting the deoxidation of sugar or glycation. If you currently take a B Complex, I suggest consider switching to the activated form of all these B vitamins.

Tip #2 – Collagen Protective Vitamins

Probably two of the most common anti-oxidants Vitamin C and E have been shown to prevent the formation of AGEs and crosslinks in collagen.

A 2002 study by Abdel et al. demonstrated an 80% decrease in glycation and AGE formation in patients supplemented with high dose Vitamin C.

Recommended Vit C dosage is 1000mg/day

Another supplement that is highly collagen protective is L-lysine.

L-lysine is an essential amino acid that means the body cannot produce it. L-lysine plays an important role in the protection and integration of collagen.

By blocking the enzyme that forms AGEs, L-lysine helps to prevent the formation of non-enzymatic crosslinks.

Although most people get an adequate amount of L-lysine from their diet, athletes, vegetarians / vegans, post-surgical or those with connective tissue injury can benefit from supplementation.

Recommended L-lysine dosage is 500mg / day

Tip #3 - An aspirin a day keeps crosslinks away

Not only is baby aspirin heart healthy, but also now studies have shown that daily aspirin can actually offset the formation of collagen crosslinks.

Aspirin inhibits the formation of AGEs by acetylating lysine residues (L-lysine + sugar = AGEs). Please note that you should not start taking aspirin daily unless you speak to your medical doctor. Those who are on blood thinners such as Plavix should not start an aspirin regimen.

Recommended aspirin dosage is 81mg / day

So we know fascial and connective tissue is key for years of movement longevity. But what do you do if you are experiencing any type of connective tissue injury that is impairing your ability to load and unload impact forces?

Considering collagen composition during your treatment or rehab protocol is important to the success of your recovery.

Considering Collagen Composition & Injury

As a Podiatrist one of the most common conditions
we treat is heel pain.

Whether it is Achilles tendonitis or plantar fasciitis
the success of patient recovery is highly dependent on
the duration of their symptoms and the health of the
connective tissue associated.

Although I wish every patient presented to my office
at the initial onset of symptoms unfortunately this is
usually not the case.

The average patient often presents after experiencing
heel pain for 3 months, 6 months or sometimes even
over a year.

The patient may have tried the occasional over the
counter insert, a little stretching and maybe even
icing, however their lack of consistency has provided
little relief.

One of the biggest misconceptions among patients is
regarding how connective tissue gets injured and the
consideration of collagen health in soft tissue
recovery.

A person can correct the muscle imbalances and
movement patterns however attention must still be
directed at the injured connective tissue and collagen
structure.

We are going to focus primarily on the connective tissue of the foot, as it is uniquely associated with a majority of impact forces during closed chain movements.

Acute vs. Chronic Injury

With each step we take 1 -1.5 x our body weight in impact forces is entering the foot and body.

Perceived as vibrations that are damped (absorbed) through isometric contractions, these impact forces are stored as potential energy in our connective tissue (tendons, fascia).

To properly absorb and store impact forces as energy our connective tissue must be under a state of tension and have a certain degree of elasticity.

I often associated our connective tissue to a rubber band. When we load impact forces and store them as potential energy this would be equivalent to stretching the rubber band.

When we do not have tensile stiffness and elasticity in our connective tissue this would be analogous to a dried out rubber band.

When you load the dried out rubber band you eventually reach a "fatigue point" and the rubber band breaks.

This is analogous to our connective tissue micro-tearing or even rupturing at a certain fatigue point.

Micro-Trauma Cycle

We explained this concept earlier, however due to the complexity of this process we will review it again in more detail.

Micro-tears in fitness are often associated with the overload principle, strength gains and muscle hypertrophy.

When we strength train (especially when doing eccentrics) we micro-tear the muscle fibers which are repaired, creating larger muscle fibers. All positives. However with connective tissue it's not so positive.

In connective tissue (tendons / fascia) when there is not enough elasticity in the tissue, micro-tears occur.

These connective tissue micro-tears are repaired with a different type of collagen than what the connective tissue is primarily composed of (Type III vs. Type I).

Type III collagen is stiffer and less elastic then Type I collagen and is laid down in a haphazard manner. In addition, all micro-tears, whether it is in muscle or connective tissue are associated with inflammation.

Persistent inflammation around connective tissue whether it be bone or tendon creates thinning of tissue.

This micro-tear, inflammatory cycle which begins as an acute stress to the tissue now becomes a perpetual cycle and we start to hit a road block in the tissue repair process.

The longer the patient's connective tissue sits in this micro-tear / inflammatory cycle, the more the tissue begins to change composition and the harder it is to establish any long lasting pain relief.

Enter chronic tendon pain.

These are the patients who do not respond to just muscle balancing and corrective exercise. Something has to be done to repair the health of the connective tissue.

So what can this patient with chronic connective tissue pain do?

Two-Step Recovery Process

Whether I am treating acute or chronic tendon pain I approach tissue recovery in two steps:

1st – Restore Connective Tissue Health
2nd – Correct Muscle Imbalances

For connective tissue health if the patient is in a chronic state my goal is to drop the patient's inflammation as quickly as possible.

Although corticosteroid injections are of great debate with conflicting research, I have seen the greatest and fastest results when I incorporate them into my patient recovery.

I am quick to give injections in my acute patients to get them out of this inflammatory cycle and have had great success with this approach.

Inflammation is like a roadblock that prevents further tissue repair and recovery.

Being able to drop the inflammatory process and allow the tissue to move forward in the repair process is a necessary step.

If steroid injections are not your cup of tea there are other options that are also available including:
- oral anti-inflammatories (my go-to is Mobic)
- topical anti-inflammatories
- ice (I never only do ice)
- Class IV laser
- Supplements such as bromelain, quercetin
- Eating pineapples or tart cherry juice

If you are not in the acute state and have had pain for greater than 6 months then the above options may not be as effective.

The longer the chronic state of tissue injury, the harder it is to bring it back to its youthful state.

In the patient that is not responding to anti-inflammatory treatment then we need to consider other options to get the connective tissue back to it's youthful, pre-injury state.

This is where we start to consider:

- PRP (platelet rich plasma)
- Bone marrow aspirate
- Amniotic membrane or
- Procedures such as Tenex and Topaz

The way that the above procedures work is by creating fresh tissue injury and restarting the inflammatory / injury cascade.

The above procedures must be followed by limited activity / immobilization and no NSAIDs can be taken during the repair process.

Once the connective tissue is returned to a more healthy state then it is time to start focusing on the muscle imbalances and compensations being placed on the connective tissue.

This is where the integration of barefoot training begins and the re-training of how to load and unload impact forces from the ground up.

In the next chapter will explore the different barefoot training programs to ensure years of movement longevity.

7 | BECOMING BAREFOOT STRONG

Now that we've thoroughly established the important role the foot plays in every closed chain movement it is time to start unleashing the power behind the barefoot.

Whether you are trying to get out of pain, improve your performance or simply looking to maintain healthy movement patterns you will benefit from the below program.

As you begin to transition into a barefoot strong lifestyle remember that little changes done daily add up to a big impact on life. The ultimate goal of becoming barefoot strong is helping you ensure years a youthful movement.

Should you be wearing orthotics?

As a barefoot friendly Podiatrist I take a non-conventional approach towards orthotics and orthopedic footwear.

The orthotic industry as a whole has gone a little out of control with thousands if unnecessary orthotics being prescribed every year.

Yes, many people do benefit from orthotics but we must remember that our foot was designed to support itself without orthotics and supportive footwear. We have become an overly supported society that is now full of lazy feet that are now dependent on these devices to function properly.

So how can you determine if you need orthotics?

Some of the most common conditions treated with orthotics include flat feet, Achilles tendonitis and bunions. But what's amazing is that these are also the most common conditions that benefit the greatest from barefoot training!

It's really a matter of how you want to approach functional movement. I always take the more holistic approach as it taps into how our body actual controls movement.

So if you currently wear orthotics or were prescribed them from a Podiatrist and are curious whether you really need them or - not ask yourself the following questions:

Do you have flat feet?

If you do have flat feet do you also have foot, knee or back pain?

If you do have flat feet but are not in pain did you ever have foot, knee or back pain for which the orthotics was prescribed?

If you do have flat feet and sometimes do not wear your orthotics or forget them how do you feel? Are you in pain? Do you feel better with or without the orthotics?

The above questions are not designed to treat or diagnose whether or not you should be in orthotics but rather get you to start thinking about why you were prescribed orthotics in the first place.

If you do not have flat feet or do have flat feet but are not in pain or never had pain associated with your flat feet - perhaps you may want to re-consider the orthotics and take a more holistic, functional approach toward ensuring proper movement.

Not all flat feet require the control or support from a custom orthotic.

So we spoke about the flat foot but what about the high arched foot?

Very rarely do I like to put this foot type in a rigid device - reason being is that this foot type already is structurally rigid.

Where orthotics are beneficial in a high arched foot is to offset pressure distribution.

In the patient that's standing on a very rigid foot evident by calluses on the 1st & 5th metatarsal head, an accommodative orthotic with dispersion area can work wonders.

Having said that, if you have a high arched foot and do not have pain or never have experienced pain then just like that flat foot I would begin to ask yourself if orthotics really are appropriate for you.

A high arched foot may benefit from an accommodative orthotic to offset pressure.

So what about the runners and athletes who were given orthotics just for their activities?

If this describes your situation then you will want to ask yourself the same questions above.

By applying the below barefoot strong concepts I have helped thousands of patients, athletes and clients from all over the world get out if their orthotics and finally be pain-free by simply tapping into their nervous system in a way it was designed to be used.

Let's continue exploring how this barefoot concept may benefit you.

Surfaces & Barefoot Training

So you are ready to embark on your barefoot strong journey but not quite sure *where* you should be doing these exercises.

The surface on which you perform the below exercises is actually much more important than you think.

If you remember in Chapter 2 we described the small nerves that are found on the bottom of the foot.

Most of the feedback used to balance and maintain stability comes from the bottom of the foot which means we want to get as much surface to foot contact as possible.

Any yoga mat, Bosu, Airex pad actually blocks the plantar receptors and is essentially just like putting your shoes back on.

The ideal surface for barefoot training is one that is hard, flat, possibly has a texture and transmits vibrations.

In 2015 my company EBFA will be releasing a special surface designed specifically for barefoot training. For more information please visit www.ebfafitness.com

The ideal surface for barefoot training is flat, stable, has a texture and transmits vibrations.

It is time to start getting barefoot strong!

The Barefoot Strong Program can be broken down into three parts: Foot Specific Programming, Foot to Core Sequencing and finally Total Body Integration.

Phase 1. Foot-Specific Programming

1. Foot Flexibility

Flexibility is always the foundation to optimal foot function.

By flexibility we mean having the adequate range of motion to function properly without compensation patterns.

Note that we did not say flexible meaning unstable or hypermobile. This means that a flat foot that is typically associated with hypermobility still often has flexibility or range of motion issues – especially in the ankle and great toe joint.

For foot flexibility I prefer to take the approach of myofascial work instead of stretching for the reasons that were mentioned in Chapter 2 and 6.

Remember more of our joint flexibility lies within fascial tissues versus actual muscle fiber flexibility.

Plantar foot release

Start by releasing the bottom of the foot with a golf ball, tennis ball or stick.

I am not partial to any of the foot massage products on the market but if you have a preference please feel free to use any product you like.

The key to the plantar foot release is to not roll on the ball. Stand in various areas on the bottom, shifting to a new area every minute.

If releasing both feet is too intense then do one foot at a time. You can even do it seated to control the amount of pressure on the foot.

Release the bottom of the foot for 5 minutes every morning, evening and before working out.

After releasing the plantar foot shift your attention to the lower leg.

For at least 5 minutes release the back of the calf (soleus), the front of the shin (tibialis anterior) and the side of the lower leg (peroneals).

Again I am not partial to any special roller but if you have a brand you like please use your preferred product.

Step 2. Foot Strength

After releasing the foot it is time to activate the intrinsic muscles in the bottom of the foot. In Chapter 2 we discussed Short Foot.

This is the go-to exercise for barefoot strength and will be the way we integrate foot to core sequencing.

Activating Short Foot

To perform short foot exercise start by standing *barefoot* on both feet, but focus your attention on one foot at a time.

Find your foot tripod that is under your 1st metatarsal head, 5th metatarsal head and heel. Lift your toes, spread them out and place them back down onto the ground.

Notice the even body weight distribution under your foot and how it feels to be in full contact with the ground. There is an energy that comes from the floor that you can feel when you are in full contact with the ground.

To activate short foot push the tip of your big toe down into the ground. If toes 2 – 5 also push down that is okay. As you push the big toe down into the ground you should feel the muscles of the arch engage. Begin to notice the ball of your foot lifting off of the ground and an increase in your arch.

Hold short foot for 10 seconds before releasing and trying it on the other foot. To see a video demonstration of how to perform short foot please visit www.barefootstrong.com

Engage short foot 10 seconds x 5 repetitions per foot every morning or before working out.

Another great exercise for barefoot strength is called *toe-spread out*. A study actually compared this exercise to short foot and found high abductor hallucis activation in toe spread out!

Toe Spread Out

To perform toe spread out begin by sitting or standing with your foot straight. Lift the toes and spread them out as much as you can.

Focusing on just the great toe you are going to tap the floor but try to abduct the great toe when tapping. For a video demonstration on this exercise please visit www.barefootstrong.com

Perform 10 repetitions per foot x 3 sets.

The final exercise I recommend to my patients for building barefoot strength is barefoot balancing. The muscles in the bottom of the foot play an important role in single leg stability so simply standing on one foot activates these small muscles.

Barefoot Balance Training

Start by standing barefoot on one leg. Try to keep a slight flexion in the knee as this increases your instability requiring the nerves and muscles to activate more.

If balance is a concern you can start by holding onto a wall or chair and then begin to progress as you feel more comfortable.

Balance on one leg 30 seconds per side x 3 sets every morning.

Phase 2. Foot to Core Sequencing

After strengthening the foot in isolation we want to begin to integrate it's strength with the rest of the body starting with the core.

To get the best results from foot to core sequencing we want to first mobilize and activate the hip and core - similar to how we isolated the foot.

Step 1. Hip Flexibility

Flexibility of the hip and pelvis is important for achieving proper alignment and optimal muscle activation patterns.

Because the feet and hips are so closely related you always want to consider their function together. If a person has tight feet and ankles they typically present with restricted hip mobility. Similarly if someone has flat feet that are unstable, the hips are typically unstable as well.

Myofascially Release the Hips

For proper balancing of the hips and pelvis focus on the anterior hip muscles, namely the adductors, rectus femoris and tensor fascia latae (TFL).

When doing myofascial release work, I like to do cross friction massage to the muscle using a foam roller. You want to spend at least 5 minutes releasing per leg.

In an inverted foot type I also recommend doing myofascial release to the piriformis and gluteus medius muscles.

To properly release these muscles you want to switch from a foam roller and to a trigger point ball or tennis ball.

Again 5 minutes should be spent releasing the glutes and piriformis muscles. For video demonstration on how to do the above release work please visit www.barefootstrong.com

Release the anterior hip and glutes 5 min per side at least 3 times a week and before working out.

Step 2. Hip and Core Activation

After releasing the hip you want to activate the pelvic floor. Due to its important myofascial connections the integrity of this often overlooked muscle is important.

Pelvic Floor Activation

Start by lying on your back with your knees bent and your feet flat on the ground. Find a neutral spine and pelvis position.

From here you want to imagine that your pelvic floor is like the face of a clock with 12 o'clock at your pubic symphysis, 6 o'clock at your tailbone, 3 o'clock at your right hip and 9 o'clock at your left hip.

Using your pelvic floor muscles imagine drawing 12 o'clock to 6 o'clock and 3 o'clock to 9 o'clock. After drawing in the 4 corners of the clock you want to then imagine purse stringing or lifting the pelvic floor up.

The sensation when doing this properly is similar to how it feels when you stop the flow of urine. I try not to cue it as a hard kegel type exercise as this leads to over-activation and sometimes spasm in some people.

Hold each repetition for 10 seconds x 5 sets.
Do 3 times a week and before working out.

The next activation that is especially important for the flat foot individual is to the hip external rotators. Studies have shown that 6 weeks of hip external rotator strengthening can pull a STJ out of eversion and into neutral!

Hip External Rotator Activation

Describing this exercise set up can be a little confusion so for video demonstration of this exercise please visit www.barefootstrong.com

You want to begin by lying on your side with your hips stacked. Bring your bottom leg forward, flex the knee to a 90 degree angle.

Shift your top leg back and also bend the knee to 90 degrees. You may want to prop it up on a yoga block or mat to keep the hip stacked.

Focusing on just the front, bottom leg you want to externally rotate the hip by lifting the foot up. Keep the knee on the ground while externally rotating the hip.

Lift and hold for 10 secs before releasing x 5 reps per side. Do 3 x a week and before working out.

Step 3. Barefoot Balance Training

Once you mobilize and activate the hip and core it is now time to integrate the foot activation with core stability.

This is through a method called *barefoot balance training* that was briefly explained in Chapter 1. Most of the foot to core sequencing I integrate into patient or client programming is done on one leg, as this is a very functional position.

This single leg stance is the most functional position of walking, running, climbing and therefore it is important to integrate it into the nervous system to ensure movement longevity.

Barefoot Balance Training

For a video of the barefoot balance training sequences please visit www.barefootstrong.com Start by standing on one leg with the knee slightly bent. If you initially want to hold onto a wall or chair for stability you can however the goal is to eventually move away from this outside assistance.

Find your foot tripod, lift the digits and place them back down on the ground. Before engaging short foot, begin to activate the pelvic floor.

Hold short foot for 10 seconds while focusing on the deep hip and pelvic floor. As you engage short foot you should start to feel muscles firing in the hip and core.

Release and repeat on the other side.

Next progress to a small single leg squat or knee flexion. On the bottom of the squat lock in short foot, engage the core and press out of the squat.

With each squat repetition you should feel the connection between foot strength and core stability becoming stronger.

Repeat 6 – 8 repetitions per side.

The next exercise is a single leg deadlift. As you shift forward into the deadlift or hip hinge trying to keep proper body alignment.

On the bottom of the deadlift, lock in short foot, engage your core and press out of the deadlift.

Repeat 6 – 8 repetitions per side.

You want to do a 5 – 10 minutes series of barefoot balance training exercises at least 3 times a week and before working out.

The most important thing to remember when doing these exercises is that short foot is engaged on the bottom of each squat, lunge, deadlift etc.

The purpose of these exercises is to establish muscle activation patterns for reflexive stability and movement longevity.

The full series of exercises can be found on www.barefoostrong.com

Perform 5 – 10 minutes of barefoot balance training 3x a week or before working out.

Phase 3. Total Body Integration

The final phase of the Barefoot Strong Program is *total body integration.* This means that we are interconnecting the foot strength and core stability to upper body power.

By training barefoot total body integration you will note improved joint alignment, faster stability and enhanced performance which translates to all sports and activities.

Step 1. Shoulder Flexibility

Just as flexibility was the foundation to our foot function and core stability, it is also the foundation to function in the upper body.

Again we are going to use myofascial release as the go-to flexibility method. For the upper body one of the most restricted and over-recruited muscles is the pectoralis.

Myofascially Release the Pecs

To release the pecs you want to use a tennis ball or trigger point release ball. Now there are a couple ways in which this can be done but I prefer the method of lying on the ground to release.

Start by lying on your stomach; place the ball just medial to your shoulder joint onto your pec muscle.

Place the same arm out to the side with the elbow bent 90 degrees.

While keeping the ball on the pec muscle slowing begin to slide the arm above the head and back to the 90 degree angle.

Release for 30 secs and repeat on the other side. Do at least 3x a week or before working out.

For a video demonstration please visit www.barefootstrong.com

Step 2. Shoulder Activation

After shoulder mobilization we want to activate the shoulder stabilizers. For this we want to be in a pushup plank position.

Start with the shoulders directly over the elbows and over the wrists. Before lifting to your plank position, rotate the elbows so that the crease of the elbow faces forward. As you do this you should feel your shoulders begin to depress or stabilize.

Focusing on the hand to shoulder stability lift into the full pushup plank. Keeping the elbows rotated forward and the shoulder blades down the back, hold for 10 seconds.

This plank should be more about upper body activation versus core strengthening – although they both are ultimately connected.

Next move the hands into a diamond pushup position. Assume the same elbow rotation and shoulder stabilization before lifting into the pushup plank.

Again hold 10 seconds and release.

The final shoulder exercise would be shifting the hands wider than shoulder width. Assume the same position and hold 10 seconds.

Shoulder activation should be done 3x a week or before working out.

Step 3. Barefoot Body Tension

The final step in total body integration is building barefoot body tension.

Body tension is a concept that you may not know by name but probably already integrate into your practice.

This common term within gymnastics means that the tension of what area of the body is added to the tension of another part thereby increasing the amount of force that can be generated by the body.

Body tension follows fascial lines and the concept of tensegrity. The more tension created by the body the faster you can stabilize joints, generate force and improve performance.

To build barefoot body tension and total body integration you can do a variety of your favorite upper body exercises but for this example we will do a single leg military press.

Start by standing on one leg with the knee slightly bent and proper upper body alignment. With the weights out to the side at 90 degrees you are going to push the weights into a military press at the same time as engaging short foot and the core.

Relax the foot as you return the weights to the start position and repeat 8 times per leg.

Additional total body exercises can be performed this way including reardelt rows, kettle bell swings, lateral shoulder raise. The trick is the integration between foot, core and scapular stabilization.

For additional exercises integrating total body integration please visit www.barefootstrong.com

Advanced Application of Barefoot Training

The benefits of barefoot training far exceeds that mentioned above. One of my favorite aspects of traveling and teaching these barefoot training concepts is to hear how other professionals apply the concepts.

I've had body builders integrate barefoot activation to improve their muscle recruitment and overall definition.

I've had martial artists apply the method for faster footwork. I've had practitioners change lives by improving mobility and stability in patients with neurological injury.

The applications really are endless.

My ultimate goal with the barefoot training methodology is to positively impact lives by teaching professionals and patients the power of tapping into their nervous system.

Although we spoke primarily about the corrective exercise applications, barefoot training can be applied to almost every exercise you perform.

Next time you do box jumps or hack squats, integrate short foot and the foot to core sequencing we explored within this book.

Next time you do kettle bell swings or military presses, integrate short foot and the foot to core sequencing we explored within this book.

Understand the way the body was designed to stabilize – from the ground up - and then integrate that into your programming and lifestyle.

The nervous system is a very powerful system that can restore homeostasis throughout our movement system if given the opportunity.

Barefoot Strong Pearls

As you begin to integrate these from the ground up principles into your lifestyle remember that consistency is important.

Start by integrating these simple methods into how you start your day and how you warm-up for your workout. From there, slowly build off of the stability and strength experienced from the barefoot activation.

As you begin your barefoot strong lifestyle there are a few *Barefoot Strong Pearls* to remember:

- *Remember foot type!*

  Subtle differences exist between the different foot types and their baseline function. Some feet need to focus on recovery while others need to focus more on stability. Understanding your foot type is the foundation to this program.

- *Healthy connective tissue starts from the inside out!*

  Just like they say beauty starts from the inside out, so does our movement longevity. Remember the negative impact that uncontrolled blood sugar has on our nerves and connective tissue. Consider integrating some of the nerve protective supplements into your lifestyle and always remember to stay hydrated!

- *Youthful movement requires daily barefoot stimulation!*

The damaging effects of footwear and unnatural surfaces is a reality in today's society however by integrating daily barefoot stimulation and foot recovery you can avoid unnecessary injury.

As I leave you to explore the power of barefoot training and from the ground up programming I encourage you to have fun and enjoy this natural method of movement.

Compare the differences you feel between barefoot and shod and make a decision for yourself which you prefer. Remember that your movement and health is ultimately under your control.

Take these simple steps now to ensure years of movement longevity and unlock the power of barefoot activation.

Are you ready to become barefoot strong?

BIBLIOGRAPHY

1. DiStefano, L. Gluteal muscle activation during common therapeutic exercises. J Ortho & Sports Physical Therapy, 2009. 39(7): 532:540.

2. Geraci, MC. Evidence-based treatment of hip and pelvis injuries in runners. Phys Med Rehabil Clin N Am, 2005. 16(3): 711-47.

3. Guiliani, J. Barefoot-simulating footwear and associated with metatarsal stress injury in 2 runners. Orthopedics, 2011. 34(7): 320-323.

4. Ireland, M. et al. Hip strength in females with and without patellofemoral pain. JOSPT, 2003. 33(11): 671-676.

5. Lieberman, DE et al. Foot strike patterns and collision forces in habitually barefoot versus shod runners. Nature, 2010. 463(7280): 531-535.

6. Madhavan, S. et al. Movement accuracy changes muscle activation strategies in female subjects during a novel single-leg weight-bearing task. J Injury Function & Rehab, 2009. 1(4): 319-328.

7. McPoil, T.G. et al. Relationship between neutral subtalar joint position and pattern of rearfoot motion during walking. Foot and Ankle, 1994. 115, 141-145.

8. Nawoczenski, D. The effect of foot structure on the three-dimensional kinematic coupling behavior of leg and rearfoot. Phys Therapy, 1998. 78(4): 404-416.

9. Nilsson, J. Ground reaction forces at different speeds of human walking and running. Acta Physiol Scand, 1989. 136(2): 217-227.

10. Robbins, S. Running-related injury prevention through innate impact-moderating behavior. Medicine and Science in Sports and Exercise, 1989. 21(2): 130-137.

11. Robbins, S. Sensory attenuation induced by modern athletic footwear. J Testing and Evaluation, 1988. July: 412-416

12. Robbins, S. Running-related injury prevention through barefoot adaptations. Med Sci Sports Med, 1987. 19(2): 148-156.

13. Sekizawa, K. Effects of shoe sole thickness on joint position sense. Gait & Posture, 2001. 13(3): 221-228.

14. Snyder, K. et al. Resistance training is accompanied by increases in hip strength and change in lower extremity biomechanics during running. Clin Biomech, 2007. 24- 26-34.

15. Tiberio, D. The effect of excessive subtalar joint pronation on patellofemoral mechanics: a theoretical model. Journal of Orthopaedic and Sports Physical Therapy, 1987. 99: 160-165.

16. Wen, Dennis. Risk factors for overuse injuries in runners. Current sports medicine reports, 2007. 6(5): 307-313.

ABOUT THE AUTHOR

Dr Emily Splichal, Podiatrist and Human Movement Specialist, is the Founder of the Evidence Based Fitness Academy and Creator of the Barefoot Training Specialist®, Barefoot Rehab Specialist® and BARE® Workout Certifications for health and wellness professionals. With over 13 years in the fitness industry, Dr Splichal has dedicated her medical career towards studying postural alignment and human movement as it relates to foot function and barefoot training.

Dr Splichal actively sees patients out of her office in Manhattan, NY with a specialty in sports medicine, biomechanics and forefoot surgery. Dr Splichal takes great pride in approaching all patients through a functional approach with the integration of full biomechanical assessments and movement screens. Dr Splichal is actively involved in the correction of movement dysfunctions as it relates to sports injury and frequently performs manual therapy techniques including joint mobilization and trigger point release.

Dr Splichal is actively involved in barefoot training research and barefoot education as it relates to athletic performance, injury prevention and human movement dysfunction. Dr Splichal has presented her research and barefoot education both nationally and internationally, with her barefoot programming in over 10 countries worldwide.

Due to her unique background Dr Splichal is able to serve as a Consultant for some of the top fitness, footwear and orthotic companies including NIKE, Trigger Point Performance Therapy, Aetrex Worldwide, Crunch Fitness and Sols.